TANTRIC TOUCHES

Improve Your Health, Body, and Relationship with Erotic Tantric Massage

ZOE ZENSUAL

1001 ways of relaxing your body, mind and spirit
www.TrueRelaxations.com

the application of any of the information provided by this guide. This disclaimer applies to any damages or injury caused by the use and application, whether directly or indirectly, of any advice or information presented, whether for breach of contract, tort, negligence, personal injury, criminal intent, or under any other cause of action.

You agree to accept all risks of using the information presented inside this book. You need to consult a professional medical practitioner in order to ensure you are both able and healthy enough to participate in this program.

Table of Contents

INTRODUCTION

When you hear 'Tantra' or 'Tantric massage,' what do you think of? I'm guessing that its probably something quite exquisitely physically enticing and exotic. Some kind of practice that originates from the Asian continent that perhaps is rather unapologetically naughty. Whether one is a very sexually inclined individual or more of a chaste fella or gal, this "image" of Tantra is indeed the rather prevailing image of Tantra.

As for me, and don't ask me how and why, tantric massage raised images of smiling, jolly hippies dancing around naked around a fire, hardly touching one another while some relaxing music played softly in the background. However then I asked myself, is that all there is to it? Hippies having fun? So there and then, I decided to dive deep into the secret sensual world of Tantra.

What I've discovered is that tantric massage brings you into a mood where your thoughts and fears vanish and your sense of time thaws. You get into a state of total oblivion. Here you'll have an irresistible chance to excavate and surrender into delight and pleasure; you'll get in touch with your inmost, deepest, vital, divine, true self. Closing the door to the rest of the world, an image of beauty hails you. You enter a state of relaxation, you feel peaceful and tranquility around

1

you, your whole soul will feel a hint of that desired tantric sensuality.

The massage is extremely erotic, making sure to sooth your nerves and muscles all over your body, then offering your body and mind augmented pleasure. You'll feel the ancient spiritual arts of sanctifying a deep connection to yourself as well as to others. With the help of in-depth and deliberate breathing and visual and mental images, a physical and psychological connection is made. At the same time, you open and stimulate the Chakras, by delivering sexual energy and taking you to the route of real passion.

Your whole body, from head to toe, will surrender to the touches of your significant other or your therapist. Feeling the heat of the "others" naked body, the gentle touches of her soft skin, his deep mesmerizing stare entrancing you in the most luxurious way, and at the same time losing yourself to the most charming, adoring, cultivating, soothing, seductive touch with Tantric massage.

In this book, you will learn more about tantric massage and how it improves relations along with the other significant benefits it offers.

CHAPTER 1: TANTRIC MASSAGE EXPLAINED

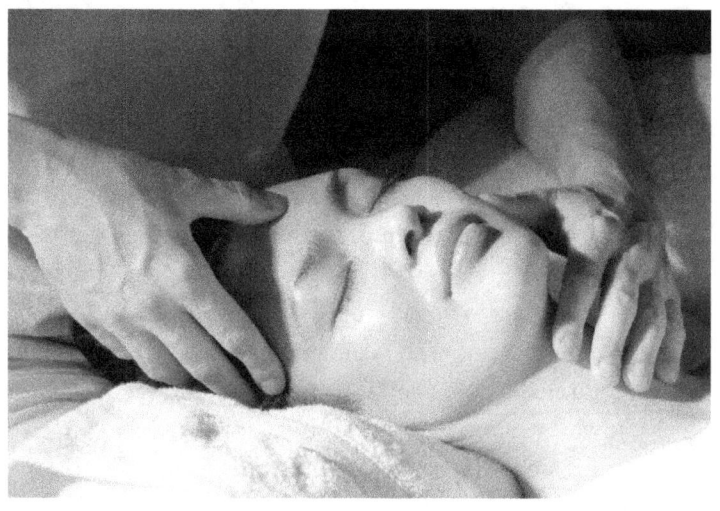

1.1 WHAT IS TANTRIC MASSAGE?

The Tantric massage is a form of sensual, erotic massage, which offers a strong theoretical and spiritual feature too. It is believed that anyone can achieve growth and satisfaction faster when he or she has an active and satisfying sex life, and even though the Tantric massage doesn't have anything to do with penetration, it can result in orgasm. You have to keep in mind that orgasm isn't the goal of the practice. Instead, it is to learn how you can stimulate and maintain the sexual energy known as Kundalini, and spread it all over the body. Another mistaken belief about tantric massage is that it comes with strict rules, processes, movements, and process that has to be followed all the time – there's nothing accurate about these things.

The truth is that the Tantric massage is a full body sensual massage which involves massaging sexual organs too, which are called Lingam (the male sexual organ) and Yoni (the female sexual organ). However, as I said, sexual satisfaction isn't the primary goal of this practice, but it is a bonus benefit. Another well-known feature of this type of massage is the desire that the giver has to get as well – since it's a very intimate process, it's normally – although not always – performed by a person with his or her partner. However, there are a lot of studios who use professionals that are incredibly talented and can offer outstanding Tantric massage too. It's essential that the giver touches the receiver in a pleasurable way as this would help them to deliver the sexual energy appropriately and bring better satisfaction. The touch and movement are also normally much milder than what are used in the traditional massage, and the feeling is that of connection and relaxation with the giver.

Another essential component of the Tantra massage is the rule that each part of the body could be touched – the Yoni and Lingam aren't the only two parts that need to be massaged as sensory receptors are located in many other parts of the body.

In order to get the whole benefits of the Tantra massage, the receiver also needs to contribute in a way that they need to learn how to trust the giver by limbering and loosening up entirely. This may sound simple, but a lot of people are having a hard time "letting go" completely as they feel susceptible throughout the sessions; this state can be overcome by tilting some of the breathing methods that could help the receiver lessen and thoroughly delight in the experience. If the two people aren't partners, they could agree ahead of time what's appropriate and comfortable for both parties.

1.2 Brief History of Tantric Massage

Many people think that tantric massage is only about sex, but the truth is that there's a lot more than that. If you want to find a tantric massage with that particular attitude, you'll be surprised at what you'll get. While sensuality and touch are a huge part of this particular style of massage, it also comes in deeper meanings that draw back to many centuries.

Tantra was essentially a type of meditative yoga that's believed to have started in India as far back as 5th century AD. The acceptance of tantric massage rapidly spread, with Asia being a continent that truly embraced this practice.

Because Asia is a big continent, it is not surprising that different versions of the massage were made in many regions. A tantric massage you will find in Japan might be completely different than the one you may find in China, just because every region has revised its own set of methods and ideologies.

The corporeal feature of tantric massage has become more popular as this practice made its way to the western world. This is maybe because that part of the world wasn't quite in touch with meditation and spiritualism as other areas were. That being said, tantric massage was normally used as a therapeutic method, particularly on women who are believed not to be too sensual.

While tantric and sensual massage is not entirely the same, they've merged today in a way that makes the tantric massage practice good for both body and mind. If you'd like to experience the pleasures of an outcall massage service, you may first ask what kind of techniques they're using. Depending on the approaches used, you may get a different experience.

How Tantra Started in the West

Tantra reached America in the year 1989 when Margot Anand published her book called The Art of Sexual Ecstasy. But even before this, Tantra has already been a common word in the west. There were writers and workshop leaders who had been excavating Eastern spiritual and sexual methods and mixing them with fundamentals of western psychotherapy, sexology, and modern self-transformational methods. One of them was Charles Muir, a yoga instructor who had followed Swami Satchidananda until he became disenchanted by the revelations of Satchidananda's unlawful sexual relations with some of the devotees. He then dedicated his time being Swami Satyananda's student, and as an instructor in the tradition of TV yoga expert Richard Hittleman.

After getting married, Muir started to retrace his methods of connecting with women. Muir also studied the ancient Tantric scriptures and began to include more and more such lessons in his yoga workshops. By the year 1980, Muir made a permanent switch from hatha yoga teacher to tantric sexuality instructor. And today, after many years, he and his wife Caroline are still undoubtedly the most famous instructors of Western Tantra.

1.3 WHO CAN LEARN AND PERFORM TANTRIC MASSAGE?

Although the real tantric methods and fundamentals may take years for anyone to master, it is still possible for you to quickly learn how to do this type of massage with your partner, especially if you're lead by a therapist. In most cases, the sessions begin with short breathing movements, staring, or conception, which prepares both receiver and giver and harmonizes their energies. Then, the conference is followed by what's basically a full body erotic or sensual massage, which integrates the touching of the female or male sexual organs. Massaging the sexual organs doesn't necessarily need to attain orgasm, but the Yoni and Lingam massages are used so as to help the receiver unclog his or her sexual tension and achieve the state of pleasure. If an orgasm is attained during the process, it's impeccably reasonable, but every session has to be approached without any fixed rules or expectation for the process to be efficient.

Just like most forms of massage, preparing the tolerable atmosphere is extremely recommended, and oils and candles are almost an essential part of every session. Sometimes, making use of flower petals or soft fabric could be a great addition and playing beautiful music would bring a good mood. During the process, the receiver has to be taken to a state of sexual stimulation, which is also a perfect way for men to learn how they can have full control of their ejaculation and for women, in order to entirely surrender and enjoy the moment of being touched.

Is Tantric Massage Only For Dissatisfied Couples?

Sexual displeasure doesn't only motivate couples who are exploring a deliberately spiritual approach to sex. A lot of them already have good sex lives, but believe that sex and relationship have the chance to give them a deeper connection and make their relationship stronger. Some couples start searching for sacred sexuality after experiencing meditation tradition from the East.

Although tantric massage help dissatisfied couples regain the fire of their relationship, many couples perform tantric massage mainly for the benefits it offers, both physically and psychologically.

1.4 What Happens During The Process Of Tantric Massage?

1.4.1 Effects for Women

Tantric massage offers the woman the opportunity to receive body touch including genitals, but without the requirement to reach orgasm. The only way to go for them is to give in and surrender themselves.

Woman's body warms up and is indulged by soft objects, then followed by some oil-rubbing. Natural oils are used together with aromatic essential oils like cinnamon, lavender, rosewood, orange, and others. The warm oil is spread on the body and is mildly rubbed. When the body reaches the relax state, the woman is equipped to get touch also in the posterior area, but of course, all things happens after an agreement. Tantric masseurs respect agreed on boundaries. Excitement ensues. The body is nurtured by the sexual vitality and turns it into dynamic energy. The goal is a gentle brook of energy associated with feelings of "euphoria". That's why there are women who experience orgasm.

1.4.2 EFFECTS FOR MEN

A great energy is born in a male body that starts to pound the entire body. When you reach the stage when the genitals are massaged, the energy can run into the entire body and lead to experiences stronger than typical orgasm.

Male massages include three types of touch in order to open up the body, which also includes warming up and oil rubbing. The oil part is the most advanced stage of the massage and like female's, it also includes massage of the genitals. Excitement turns into deep relaxation and then turns into energy from genitals through the entire body and extends the desire before ejaculation. The massage may end in the tantric way, when a mild flow of energy is made in the body, leading to experiences different from a typical orgasm. It could also end with ordinary orgasm.

1.5 Importance of Sex and How It Improves Relationship

The secret to keeping passion and sex life active in a relationship is by focusing on things that will develop your connections with one another, which something tantric massage offers. What makes sex so passionate is the state of mind and feelings a couple offered to each other. It's so simple that a lot of people don't manage to see it. The most apparent of all the things that happen in any relationship is virtually never seen by those who are in the relationship.

There are a lot of ways to improve your sexual performance and the relationship. Remarkably though, a lot of them start out of your bedroom. The more you focus on the intimacy and the excellence of your connection together, the more blockades you can destroy in the bedroom.

Each person wants to be loved and appreciated. If you put your attention on these things throughout the times you are together; you'll notice an enormous change in the excellence of your life as a couple. When you start the humdrum of day-to-day activities, it could be easy to freeze yourself to romance. It's a critical love killer. Whenever you do something surprisingly kind, and with modified detail, the passion starts to roll in again. You could do that sort of thing, and you have to be doing this on a daily basis.

Most people have no idea just how important having good mental health is beneficial for sex.

Most of the time, sex reflects the current state of a relationship and what you can achieve is so thoroughly related to what you feel.

If you're possessed by your past or the past of your partner, then expect for the future to be dreary. You have to remember that past is past, so move on! That's possibly the best advice somebody you could follow when in relations.

These are great ingredients to keeping a relationship soulful and alive. One of the most important things is for you listen to one another, and sex is considered to be one of the best forms of communication. So, practice every type of communication, and you'll improve naturally.

Chapter 2: Three Types of Tantric Massage

There are three main types of tantric massage you can have, let us look at each of them…

#1: Individual Tantric Massage

Tanric massage involved exploring an inviolability of yourself through different parts of your body that are symbols of the divine. According to Tantra, the human body isn't really a body but instead, manifestations of human polarities.

Visualization and vibrations of sound, body, and breath help stimulate and invigorate your sensual and physical body vitalities and recombine with the eternal part of you that goes throughout your body. It is an intimate experience that runs beyond the meaning of physical affection; it is about self-Intimacy intimacy.

#2: Sacred Spot Massage

This type of tantric massage is a far-fetched experience that really promotes self-loving by accepting and appreciating everything around you at the moment.

Most of the time, there's an experience curve that receivers usually experience while under a Sacred Spot Massage. A phase of nervousness for first-timers, an expectation phase for those who have already experienced it followed by an erotic period, which is excelled into total acceptance and bliss where it is no longer only a sensual experience, but, a genuine of ecstasy, an euphoric, trance-like place of construction of body, spirit, and sex.

#3 COUPLE OR PARTNER MASSAGE

A couple or partner tantric massage is where you create, reconnect, and even relearn healthy relationship with your partner. This massage involves representing clear, intensely honest message, boundary exploration, limitation setting, and recreation, similar to a Tantra Partner Session, however, here you make use of massage and sensual mindfulness methods, and it is apparently making use of the body as the truck for connection.

During this massage, you and your partner are able to explore sensitive touch from your partner's viewpoint as you get to listen not only with your ears but as well as your heart and body. There might be new consciousness of your own sexual expression that can dig out your connection, with your partner as well as yourself.

CHAPTER 3: HEALTH BENEFITS OF TANTRIC MASSAGE

The benefits offered by Tantric massage based on the belief that both physical and spiritual have to live in harmony and the only way for us to live our life to the fullest is to achieving that balance. The massage is also derived from the belief that massaging the entire body is the only means to stimulate our senses and ward off our worries and frustrations.

As mentioned earlier, one of the biggest misconceptions about tantric massage is that is all about giving sexual pleasure or to help the receiver learn how to lengthen sexual pleasure – although both of these elements are parts of the session, they're just a hailed part of the entire process and in no way its objective. The primary goal is to carry sexual energy properly, which is very powerful, and use it as a tool for positive self-realization and self-progress. For us to be successful in our career, social, and personal life, it is necessary for us to free ourselves from unnecessary burdens, negative thoughts, sexual frustration, and bad relationship; these things are only some of the areas, where the Tantric massage are able to help.

There are a lot of benefits offered by Tantric massage, as documented by the ancient sadhus and rishis of India who developed this art and the earliest implementers too. Below we listed down these benefits and you'll see

16

how they're quite helpful and essential in the modern world we live in

Complete Physical Surrender

A tantric massage session teaches you to entirely surrender yourself and body to your partner while getting what could be the best sensation you've ever gotten. This form of submission is unattainable in our money-oriented life. It's safe to say that a Tantric massage is beneficial in unraveling your spiritual self from within.

Better Health

The tantric massage improves your circulation, emotional health, and reduces stress. Each of these leaves you in improved wellbeing, with a better emotional and physical attitude going forward.

Emotional Healing

Tantric is most importantly targets your emotional health. While there are delightful physical aspects, you are able to expect even better results when it comes to your emotions. As you start learning to experience pleasure, self-worth, and self-esteem are heightened, which leads to a better general pleasure.

Highest Level of Pleasure

Some people have experienced pleasures like an orgasm and sometimes more, through a carefully-directed Tantric massage. When performed correctly, it could also give an orgasm to those who have never done it before, particularly on women.

Become Self-Aware

There is no better way to become aware of your very self than by giving up complete control in every aspect to another person. A tantric massage requires you to abandon inhibitions and insecurities and lay them at the hands of the masseuse. As every part of your body is given complete attention, you will get to know yourself in new ways and discover parts of your inner-being that you weren't previously aware of.

Fight Stress

Any form of massage helps those who are experiencing stress, tantric massage, on the other hand, takes it to the next level and don't focus on relaxing the body alone. Because tantric focuses on your physical, spiritual emotional and sexual wellbeing simultaneously, you'll leave with a transformed sense of self and reduced stress using it.

Improvement of Libido

The idea of Tantra is general development. When the body's innermost dormant energies of are released through this practice, the libido of the person goes through a great increase. It's extremely likely that this person is going to increase performance even throughout ensuing events of regular sex.

Better Breathing   Pattern

Tantric massage involves different breathing methods that have been proven to be effective for many years. The breathing techniques you'll use throughout your massage will help to improve the general experience and furthermore teach you how to control your breath and synchronize it with the natural responses of your body.

Improved Energy and Vitality

The Tantric massage can generate constructive difference, and one of them is that the person develops in stamina. The massage can unlock parts of the body that have been chained and narrowed and can even fix the body's deterioration. Because of this, the person becomes more productive in different parts of their life.

Makes One Look and Feel Younger

If you think that you are still young, then doing Tantric massage will make you look and feel younger. Because you become sexually active even more and because you get more energy to perform your everyday activities, you no longer feel your age. You feel younger. This also gives confidence in you and improves your self-reliance.

Relax Your Body

A tantric massage relaxes a lot more than just a scoring back and shoulders. All parts of your body are precisely cared for, not a mere part of your body is ignored. A lot of first timers are amazed that they can keep very relaxed while getting stimulated simultaneously, but tantric massage pursues to please and relax your whole being at the same time.

If you're planning to have a tantric massage, the benefits are clearly much more than just helping pain or difficulty you experience in your body. You might have never undergone a lengthy feeling of stimulation. However, the result will possibly be more prevailing than you probably imagined.

CHAPTER 4: GETTING STARTED

Massage is one of the best ways to get rid of tension in the body, improve the circulation of the blood, spread energy all over the body, and sexually turn on your lover's desire! Massage is also an equally satisfying way to help couples show intimacy to each other. We, by nature, starve for touch, and massage is a fast, simple means to fulfill this needs. Sounds simple, right? Well, getting a certificate or proper training to perform tantric massage is not necessary. An essential part of a good massage is the yearning to satisfy your partner. So, here we provide you with some suggestions to get started.

4.1 PREPARING FOR THE MASSAGE

The idea of tantric massage to those who have not experienced it before is rather intriguing, if not, intimidating. On the other hand, people who are familiar with it find it unique, exciting and maybe more pleasing. The problem, however, is that not many people know what it is and how it work, so they don't even consider it.

For the perfect tantric massage, it is best for partners to take turns on massaging each other. As mentioned earlier, this type of massage requires the receiver to be vulnerable, to surrender himself or herself completely.

But of course, this massage is not just allowing the giver to do whatever he wants to do.

If you have low self-esteem or just too conscious about yourself, tantric massage will teach you how to appreciate yourself even more. It is also helpful in boosting your partner's confidence as you enjoy being near him or her and helping them feel accepted and loved. To get started, here are some preparations you have to do before starting up the process:

1. Get Your Space Ready

Prepare the bedroom or any area you want to use, may it be a living room or anywhere private, with many soft pillows and comfortable bedding. Put several lighted, but generally aromatic candles, all over the area — securely away from things that are flammable. Keep your lighting totally off or on the dimmest place.

Pour in drinking water or wine in a clear glass within reach so that it will be convenient for you. You might even want to place some light snacks in order to keep the energy up or to feed one another. If you want for the room smell good, you may want to use an essential oil diffuser with a soothing scent.

2. Prepare Yourself Physically, Mentally, And Spiritually

Before you start up, make sure that you have an open heart and an open mind. If something causes you discomfort, it is best to skip them, but if you can try to work through anything that leads you to this feeling. The most common discomfort one experiences are due to consciousness about his or her body. During the practice, keep being playful and show interest in finding new types of pleasant interaction.

Before the session starts, you may want to take a bath or shower, doing it together would be better, but avoid sexual interaction during that time. Stand up face to face and stretch nevertheless, suits you to let go any tension.

Wear comfortable clothes. Make sure that the underwear, shorts, lingerie, and shirt that loose enough for easy removal. However, doing them without wearing anything would be a great option too. But since tantra is about a slow accumulation of sexual energy, it is usually helpful to get started with your clothes on.

3. Initiate The Process By Building Sexual Energy Slowly

After doing some stretching and taking a shower, sit down facing each other and be comfortable. You might want to sit cross-legged, or place your legs over each other in order for the energy from the erogenous zones gets closed to each other.

Stare at each other for at least five minutes — it is said that the eyes are the windows to the soul, and this applies very well to this situation. You may find it uncomfortable at first, but carry on to stare at each other's eyes as long as you can. The moment you feel comfy, a connection has been built. That's the goal. That's the exact sense of connection that you need in order to revel in tantric sex. Keep your eye contact all throughout the practice.

4.2 STARTING THE TANTRIC MASSAGE

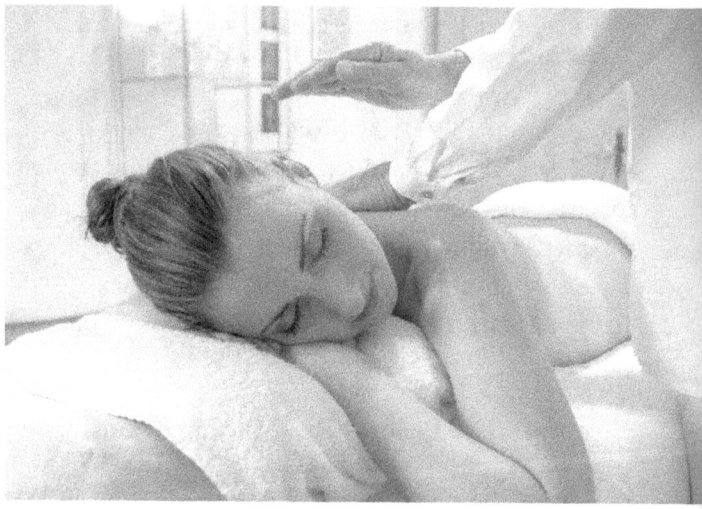

Here are simple methods you can follow. These are simple massage methods you can perform with or without experience on this practice.

Start with your Back Side

About two tablespoons of oil have to be enough to get started. Smear the oil all over your hands first and then start rubbing your hands to make your palm warm. Then put your hands on the lower back of your lover and allow your hands to slither up the back of your love throughout the neck, all over the shoulders and back, all over the buttocks area.

The Hand Slide

Now that you have got the oil on the back of your lover, start sliding your fingers down the spine, massaging throughout to the lower back and over the buttocks. Move up to the neck, then on the shoulders, and then the arms and the fingertips. Repeat it at least five times. As you perform this, communicate with your love and ask what if feels like or any feedback. If your lover is the type that doesn't talk a lot, you don't have to force him or her. Keep in mind that, it is all about giving your partner pleasure.

Pull-Ups

For a change, try changing one hand after another as you pull up and rub the side of your lover's body. Begin by putting both of your hands on his or her hips and then softly pull up to the spine.

Move your hands over the waist and pull up to the spine. Then place your hands on the side of the breast and go back to the spine. Place your hands just below the armpits and pull up to the spine. Make sure you do both sides.

Kneading

If you bake, then this method would be a piece of cake (no pun intended.) However, if you have not, you can simply squeeze your lover's back and back sides between your thumb and other fingers in a sinuous motion using one hand, and then the other. Next, glide your hands to another part on the back and do the same process over and over until your partner has been well-kneaded starting from the neck down to the buttocks. The body's fleshy parts such as the buttocks could bear more pressure, so, don't worry about squeezing it a bit harder and slightly spread the cheeks while kneading. This will surely make your partner excited.

Feather Stroke

Before moving onto the thighs, stroke the neck, arms, shoulders, back, and buttocks of your partner using your fingertips in an extremely light stroke. Do it for about five minutes. If your fingernails are long, scratch your partner's skin lightly. You are able to do this in circular motions, from side to the other. Allow for your light, prickly touches, and strokes make sensual eagerness for your lover as he wouldn't guess which part of his or her body you are going to touch next.

Foot Caress

You will perhaps need more oil on this. Add more oil on your hand, rub your hands together, and put more on your partner's body. Now, start the hand slide method on the thigh as well as the calf moving slowly. Start doing the kneading stroke again, followed by softer one. Do single leg at a time. It is worth noting that the feet are a great erogenous zone, so you have to put a considerable attention to it! Put more oil on each foot, rubbing it all over the ankle, then the heel, and in the middle of the toes. With your palms, slide on the bottom of the foot of your partner back and forth a couple of times. Rotate your partner's toes clockwise and then counter-clockwise and lastly, glide your forefinger between every toe. Softly pull every toe away from his or her body.

Turn your Lover Over

By this time, your partner is surely pleasured of what you just did on his or her back. Now, carry on by focusing on your partner's frontal area. Again, put more oil in your hands and then smear it on your lover's belly button, gradually sliding them up the core of his or her stomach and all over their nipples, then down to your partner's belly button. Do it over and over because your partner will love it and it spread energy onto his or her body. If your lover is a female, make sure to be careful when you are already on her breast. Male can bear strokes that are firmer. Actually, you can do kneading on the male's chest.

4.3 DIFFERENT TANTRIC MASSAGE POSITION

When you are finally ready to get to the next level, there are simple tantric massage positions that are perfect for beginners. Depending on your flexibility level, you are able to modify the poses based on your liking and comfort. The most important thing is to concentrate on the connection and the time you spend with your partner and enjoy the presence of each other. Hopefully, you'll experience a better bond within a calm state. Begin at your comfortable level, communicate your various levels of flexibility and strength, and most importantly, practice lengthy eye to eye contact, feeling the touch of each and positive thoughts about each other without saying a single word.

Below are some tantric poses you can try with your partner:

1. YAB YUM

This pose is beneficial in aligning energy between couples. One partner sits cross-legged on a mat comfortably. Then, the other partner sits over the thighs of the other and cross his or her ankles at the back of

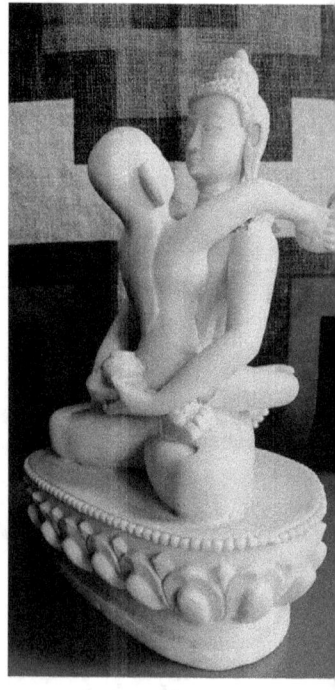

the partner. Make use of your abdominal and lower back muscles in order to keep straight and aligned with one another. Make your touched and breathe intensely and slowly consistently. You can do this pose either your eyes are closed or open.

In performing this pose, I'd recommend for you to move through these three steps to develop a safe space and to reassure energetic affection to form slowly. Every "sit" has to be 20 minutes long. Don't forget to set a timer, so you don't have to worry about the time while doing the process.

Step 1: Both of you and your partners must sit in Easy Pose facing one another with knees lightly touching. Put your hands on the knees of each other. Stare into each other's eyes without paying attention to anything in the room. Slow down your breathing pattern until your breaths synchronize. Inaudibly negotiate a breathing rhythm that you know is comfortable for both of you.

Step 2: You and your partner open up your legs. The woman must sit as close as possible to her partner, wrapping her legs around his and over his lower back. Put your hands on each other's waist or shoulders. Placing your hands on each other's heart would be an option too. Like on the first step, it's also important to watch your breathing pattern.

Step 3: The final position of this pose is the classic position shows on the image above. The woman sits entirely on the lap of her partner. Start facing each other with foreheads touching and arms comfortably around each other. At this point you should still be staring at each other's eyes; the eye contact slowly turns into increased physical touch, as you concentrate on the breathing.

Notice the quality of the energy now. What does it feel like? Where in your body do you feel it? Let it move freely. Let your bodies embrace fully. At this time, the feminine energy of the woman, as well as her creative life force and kundalini, are all developing.

2. BOAT POSE

In this pose, you will use your core muscles significantly. This is a good pose for stretching and strengthening. This is also a yoga pose that when done alone and incorrectly, it may give you lower back pain because if you do not already have the abdominal strength, the muscles at your lower back will try to keep you in good balance, but this risk is lower when done with a partner. Furthermore, you are able to modify it depending on your comfort and flexibility.

Step 1: Sit on the floor facing each other with your legs out in your front, and your knees bent a little.

Step 2: With your bent knees, move onward until and put the soles of your feet at the feet of your partner and reach each other's hands. Lean your back and thrust your feet against your partners.

Step 4: Gently unbend your legs, but at the same time, keeping your feet touching.

Step 5: In order to deepen the connection, bend your knees once again slowly, keeping your sole at its position, and then move your legs separately on both sides of. Uncurl your knees once more with your legs out of your arms.

3. DOWNWARD DOG

Now if the boat pose is not for you because you think you are not flexible enough, this one is an easier pose, which is perfect for beginners. This is one of many couples' top favorite. You will feel good arching your spine and stretching through your abs and chest at the same time as your partner. Because it involves balancing, getting in position can be a challenge, but it's easy to get it mastered.

Here is how you do it:

Step 1: Both of you begin in a tabletop position; one ahead of the other. Walk back to that position about 5 to 6 inches, tucking toes below, so your feet's balls are not touching the floor.

Step 2: As you exhale, lift your sit bones upward and carry the body into a descending V shape, so you both be in a classic downward-facing dog position.

Step 3: Walk slowly on your feet and hands back until it's easy for you to walk your feet to the outside of their lower back. Stop when you find the hips, and you can stay on the position gently.

Step 4: Communicate as your feet do the transitions in order to make sure they are not hurting and for you to keep your connection.

Step 5: Stay in that position for 5 to 7 breaths, then your partner must slowly bend his or her knees, lowering the hips until reaching tabletop position and then child's pose as you gently release feet to the ground. You can do it again swapping places.

This is a simple inversion that carries length in your spine. It is also great in improving communication and intimacy.

4. SEATED TWIST

This is a tantric massage pose where both of you have to sit cross-legged, facing one another. Spinal twists pose is known to be a really relaxing pose when done alone, but when performed with your partner, this pose could not just improve your wicked spines and sooth your overall feeling, but also can fire up intimacy.

This is how you can perform this tantric massage pose:

Step 1: Sit in a calmly seated position facing each other, your knees should touch each other.

Step 2: Sit up straight with your body a little forward, shoulders relaxed and chin pointed a little down.

Step 3: Put your left arm at your back and lengthen your other arm out. Make your partner do the same thing.

Step 4: Reach for the left hand of your partner using your right hand while you offer your left hand to the right hand of your partner. This position will twist your body which is your goal.

Step 5: Slowly twist your body for as much as you want, but make sure you both still comfortable. Keep in continuous communication throughout the process.

Step 5: Stay in this position for at least two minutes and then switch sides.

5. Forearm Stand

Forearm Stand benefits the shoulders, core, arms as well as the back, and stretches the shoulders and chest. This tantric pose also strengthens and invigorates the body, improves proprioception and balance, and develops overall blood circulation. It's a great pose to practice balance and focuses on trusting your partner.

This pose is a great practice done alone, but better when done with a partner; here is how you do it.

Step 1: Do a flanking position on the floor and kick back in the air and get your partner hold your ankles when they go high enough that your body goes into vertical position.

Step 2: when your partner have both of ankles, and you finally feel stable, ask them to put one of their fists in between of your ankles. Ask your partner to let go slowly and you must be able to stay fluctuating if you keep the hug of your inner thighs by enfolding his or her wrist.

In order to release, ask your partner to hold onto your hips, in order for you to hinge from the hips going down.

4.4 Important Tips for Performing Tantric Massage

Here are some important tips you may want to follow to make the most of the Tantric massage.

Tip #1: Perform It At Least Once A Week

Try to commit to tantric session on a regular basis with your partner. Choose a day and time that suits your schedule.

Save at least 2 hours to rejoice your connection and relationship really. Don't postpone although you feel exhausted, as your tantric massage session will soon revitalize your mind and body and make you feeling fresh and energized.

Make sure to be consistent with to your set date and only reschedule when you really need to. You will be surprised with the better connection, love, and playfulness every session brings to both of you!

Tip #2: Be Open to Try Something New

Don't forget to have fun and keep in mind that you don't have to take yourself seriously all the time. You don't only need to open your thoughts but also your heart, although something feels silly to you in the beginning.

A lot of people who haven't experienced tantric massage before have professed the eye-glazing exercise weird and awkward until they finally tried it!

Do not lay off anything, just save some practices until you are ready to try with them later. And don't forget that being playful and curious makes everything better makes everything better.

TIP #3: SET THE MOOD
You have to remember that setting is important to improve the atmosphere of the place and you can do that by cleaning and decorating your bed with soft cushions and blankets. Scatter the place with flowers, diffused essential old, light incense sticks, plus some fruits and drinks that you and your partner will both enjoy.

Light up candles – their wavering and dim light will carry charmed into the place. Play a soft, soothing music playlist. And make sure that the temperature in the room should just be to ensure your comfort.

TIP #4: TAKE A RELAXING BATH
Run a soothing bubble bath for you and your partner. Light up some candles throughout the bathroom, play relaxing music, scatter flower petals on the floor, and pour in some excellent red wine.

TIP #5: SHAKE OFF YOUR BODY
Relax your body and to let go off any tension or obstructions.

Stand up facing each other with your feet hip width away and bent knees a little. Take your time and relax your whole body from head to toe and next begin shaking your entire body for at least 5 minutes – from your arms to your hands, as well as your hips, shoulders, head, and legs, you will just love the prickling and aliveness you will experience after that!

Doing this will help your bodies feel pleasure in a much more profound, stronger way.

TIP #6: MEDITATE TOGETHER

Meditating together with the intention to clear your minds and link to your hearts would be extremely beneficial. Take a seat with your legs crossed facing one another and both eyes closed.

Take a deep breath – just be there in silence until you feel comfortable and all your worries go away. This will make you be aware of your surroundings and be fully present and engrossed to each other.

You are also able to play a directed meditation, calming music, or just sit there silently.

TIP #7: TELL YOUR PARTNER THE THINGS YOU LOVE ABOUT THEM

Look at them straight in the eye, and start every sentence with 'I love…'

Be genuine, digging deep into your heart to say everything you like about them. Keep in mind that this is about discussion and not only for the sake of discussion.

TIP #8 START THE TANTRIC MASSAGE PROCESS
Have the receiver lay facing down, as you stimulate their body to different sensations.

Touch their skin softly with fabrics, flowers, feathers, hot wax, ice, or only using your fingertips. Start with a mild touch, and then make it longer, fuller eventually. Begin at non-erogenous areas like the back, head, neck, hands, feet, and legs then gradually stimulate their sexual energy by caressing their bottom, inner thighs, and then the genitals.

Turn your partner over and do the same thing in the front – arousing them with your soft touch, and then massaging the non-erogenous parts of their body first before going up to their chest, tummy, inner thighs, and then genitals.

Ask them how it feels to get their feedback.

ENDING THE SESSION
By the end of the massage, it is up to you and your partner whether you are going to have sex or not. Otherwise, just cuddle and share passionate conversation.

If you choose to have sex, it is important not to rush it. Let the penetration to take place naturally, without exerting too much effort.

Begin with gentle, shallow thrusts, and keep totally conscious of your bodies, your vitalities, and mainly your genital region. Guide your awareness to travel all around your spine and all the sensations you feel.

And as you begin to move again, let your genitals to bond affectionately, and thaw together in a beautiful, delighted dance.

IT IS IMPORTANT TO TAKE IT SLOW

Foreplay is important in Tantra. A relaxed, slow movement helps you control longevity of women's arousal. The more you pay attention to the process of building energy, the longer the session is going to last and the more energy you'll form. Take your time to concentrate on each other entirely. Just like in meditation, when your thoughts wander, mildly guide your focus back to your partner and the process.

Conclusion

You can describe Tantric Massage as a delightful full naked body massage that starts with light touches which lead to deep strokes. Using feathers or other kinds of props could also be considered. Using relaxing music, candles, and essential oils offers the mind calm feeling to receive this particular time just to forget all the worries you have and live in the moment.

There are many other definitions of Tantric Massage in the today's modern world, all from different points of views; not all steady but definitely valid. But it's fair to say that "Tantra" is a union of old Tantric Massage methods together with sensual and traditional soothing body effort. This results in a distinctive form of amplified sensations which leads to the best intimate recreation one ever experienced.

It's not easy to explain these strong feelings even after experiencing it. Tantric massage takes over and spreads mental and physical pleasures with thoughtful, professional human physical interaction in such a sensual way.

Tantric massage is not only about touches and strokes, but also commanding conception and special breathing methods. In unison, they create a huge impact at a person's physical, emotional, and spiritual level. This form of massage comes with a lot of health benefits, which range from purely physical ones, such as immunity boost and stress relief, to emotional issue and healing of mental sufferings. This form of massage is an exceptional way to detain finer discernments of sexuality and develop healthier, stronger, and more intimate relationships between two lovers.

But that's not only about it. Tantric massage can also be the pathway to indescribable spiritual pleasure, the entry to the Numinous, which lets you pass through the limits of time and space to the sweet grip of love and harmony of the universe.

With the benefits tantric massage offers, you may think that it is overwhelming, but it is not! Anyone can do this without proper training. A lot of people from all walks of life can perform and take advantage of its benefits when done correctly.

Through tantric massage, you and your lover can start a sensual and erotic journey towards your whole body awareness, love, and intimacy. This unique form of massage done by couples opens up the mind, body, and feelings to spread sexual energy all over the body. With this ancient practice originating in India, you will not only rekindle or improve the fire of your relationship but also give your whole entity something that can't be offered by other forms of massage.

ONE LAST THING

If you liked this book, feel free to leave a review!
And if you happen to be craving more ecstasy and
healthy relaxations, make sure to visit

www.TrueRelaxations.com